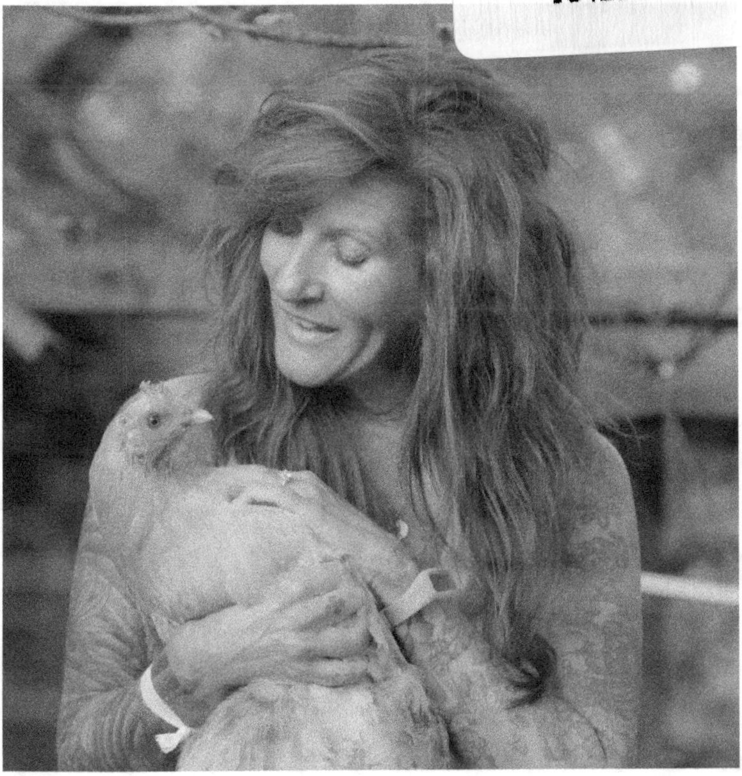

Lara Foldvari

PULSE

keep the beat of youth

Lara Foldvari

Pulse

Please note:

1. I am not a doctor (I don't even play one on TV). For anything beyond the scope of this book, please refer to the appropriate medical professional.
2. The information in this book should complement in-person nutrition and fitness coaching.
3. YoLarates™, LLC is a business trademarked by Lara Foldvari.
4. Cover photo by JL Reynolds photography
5. Copyright © 2015 by Lara Foldvari.
6. ISBN-13:978-1519436542
ISBN-10:1519436548

Thank You

To all of my students, and clients, and friends and family for letting me experiment on you!

And...

To Larry for being my first love, and to Bruce for being my last... I love you both always!

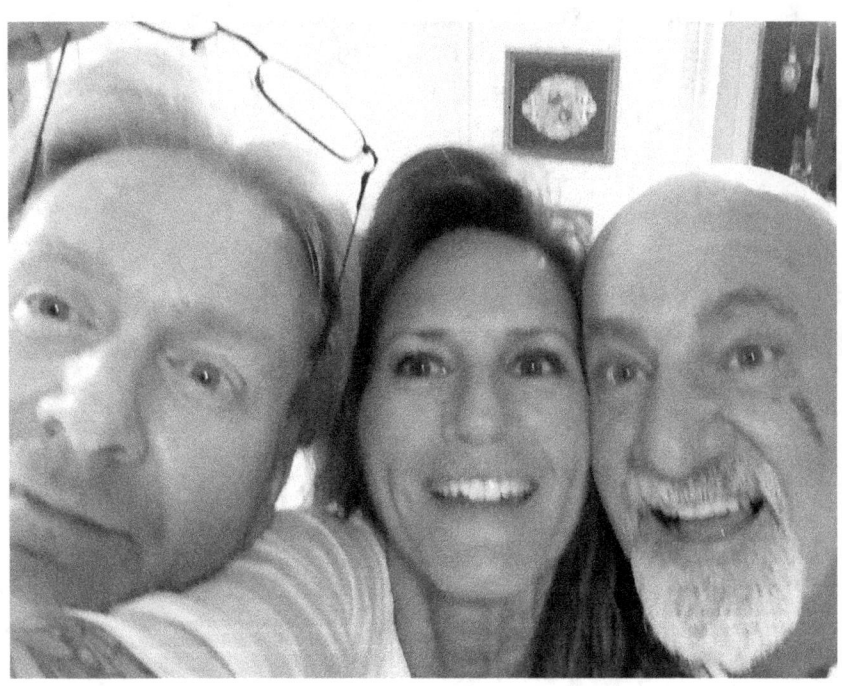

Table of Contents

Introduction..7
Pulse...11
Pulse-8 Plus...12
   1. Lentils (and other beans, AKA PULSES)...................15
   2. Avocados, olive oil, and other plant fats....................18
   2.5 Coconut Oil...20
   3. Walnuts, almonds, and other nuts (even peanuts, which are actually a legume)..21
   4. Salsa...23
   5. Eggs...24
     6. Chicken, fish, and other lean meat
....25
     7. Vegetables (leafy and other greens, plus the rest of the rainbow)...26
   8. Apples and berries and other fruits (including raisins and prunes)..28
    Plus: WINE!..30
Pulse Fast...38
Pulse Supplements 43
Pulse Exercise..45
Pulse Smoke and Mirrors..47
Pulse Lists...51
   At the grocery store:..51
   Meal Plan- what Lara typically eats on any given day....55
   Favorite recipes...57
Final Thoughts...63
Appendix I..64
   Bibliography..64
   Suggested Reading...66
Appendix II...67
   Stuff I love..67
   Beauty Products I love...67
   Favorite Apps for my iPhone.......................................67

Websites to check out 68
Appendix III..69
The 3-4-7 Cleansing Detox Jumpstart......................................69
3-day Cleanse...69
4-day Detox 71
7-day Jumpstart...73
About the Author..75

Introduction

I am 48 years old, and proud of it! I stopped lying about my age when I turned 21 and was able to legally purchase wine. What's the point?

My boyfriend is five and a half years older than me. When we got together, his friend's daughter Elizabeth said, "Bruce, why do you look 65 and your girlfriend looks 35?" Out of the mouths of babes... He does look a little older than he is (early balding and graying), and I look a little younger than I am (smoke & mirrors- more on that later), but the 35-65 stretch may be stretching it.

Although, Elizabeth isn't the only one. When we travel, TSA agents comment on how nice it is for Bruce to be taking his "daughter" on vacation with him. And a Connecticut State Trooper once stopped me for speeding, but thanked me for keeping my intoxicated "father" off the roads.

This past summer, my first boyfriend came to visit from Florida. We met when I was 11 years old and he was 16 years old. The last time I had seen him was 24 years ago. A lot can happen to a woman's face and figure in two and a half decades, and it usually isn't good.

However, when I worried out loud about being "old," Larry told me that I needed to bottle what I was doing, because I looked "terrific." And he saw me in a bikini in broad daylight poolside, and in my glasses with no make-up on, before coffee. I can't bottle it (yet), but I can tell you what I do to keep looking, and more importantly feeling, terrific.

Many of us make lifestyle changes to lose weight and look good.

And for those of us over 40, looking good often equates to looking younger. (Side note: Just the other day, I was kind of complaining about "old dudes" checking out half-naked 25 year olds. Bruce asked what my problem was with 25 year olds. "I'm not one." Luckily, he's OK with that, but society can do a job on our egos.) So yes, I am guilty of working to look younger.

But honestly, I am more concerned with feeling younger. Feeling, and being, healthier. So that I can stay "young" for decades to come.

After years of trial and error on myself, and of successes with students and clients, I believe that I have come up with a very realistic and do-able plan. My "bottle."

Its' not just diet. It's not just exercise. You've heard it before. You've even heard it from me in my book , *The exhiLarate 10-steps to a Healthier- and Happier- You.* You need to do both. Thankfully, you don't have to do too much of either to have great success. In fact, I've been embracing a less-is-more philosophy.

So, what do I do? How do I do it? What's my plan? What's in that bottle?

You may have noticed that the name of this plan is "Pulse." I decided on that for a few reasons, and for a few of the definitions of the word.

First: I eat a lot of pulses (AKA legumes or beans)
Second: My main form of exercise incorporates many pulses (little movements)
Third: This plan will help you to keep your heart pulsing for the long-run

Pulse

OK, so there's more to it than that.

I do eat a lot of pulses. On the mornings that I eat breakfast (waitwhat? Didn't she used to tell us that breakfast was the most important meal of the day and to never skip it? Yeah, more on that later.), I will have lentils, or refried beans, or black beans with my eggs. I'll throw beans into my salad at lunchtime. Often, at dinner, instead of a rice or pasta or potato, I will have beans as my starch.

I'm always looking for ways to add lean protein and fiber to my diet, and pulses cover both.

In addition to that, I try to eat a lot of vegetables. Fruit, too. The fat I eat is mostly from plants, and I try to stay away from gluten, most dairy, and sugar & processed foods.

Oh, and I drink wine. Pretty much every day.

Pulses for exercise? I created, and teach, a yoga, Pilates, ballet fusion class (barre), called YoLarates™ in which I give the instruction to pulse about a dozen times in a one-hour class. Maybe more. I try to limit my workouts to 4-5 days a week, and I keep them low-intensity and low-impact.

So what about that skipping breakfast business? Sometimes I skip lunch, too! Gasp! It's called intermittent fasting, and while it sounds like you'll be starving, you won't. It's easy, and you see results quickly.

My diet is high quality, but today's food isn't the same as yesterday's, so I do supplement. No multivitamins for me, though. Just some superfoods and collagen.

And I keep it real. 80/20. 80 percent of the time I am following this plan, and 20 percent of the time I am veering wildly off-course with a slice of pizza in one hand and a beer in the other. Life is meant to be lived, and it's not worth it if you are constantly and continuously keeping yourself from enjoying it.

Oh, and as insurance that I look as good on the outside as I feel on the inside? Smoke and mirrors, baby. Smoke. And. Mirrors.

That's it. Read on for the nitty gritty.

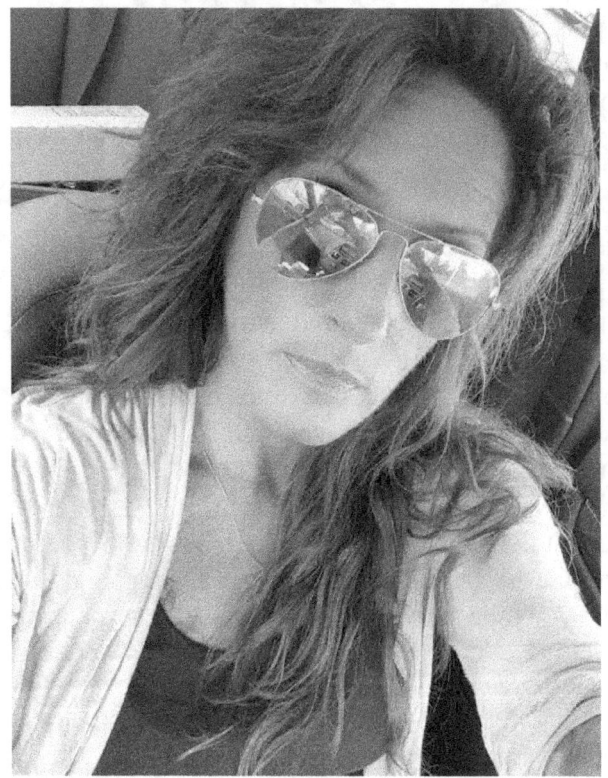

Pulse

Definition of *PULSE* from the Merriam-Webster Dictionary

noun

- the edible seeds of various crops (as peas, beans, or lentils) of the legume family

- the regular expansion of an artery caused by the ejection of blood into the arterial system by the contractions of the heart

- rhythmical beating, vibrating, or sounding

verb

- to move with strong, regular beats
- to produce a strong, regular beat
- to be filled with activity or a feeling

Pulse-8 Plus

Pulse-8. Pulsate Get it? These are the eight foods that you should eat on a regular basis (almost daily) as the basis for your weight management and vibrant vitality. I don't like to tell you what you can't eat, because putting a positive spin on things is always better. (I also don't "cheat." In my world, it's a "treat." Way better, right?) I will, however, tell you what I think you should limit to special occasions or treats.

Note: I don't think you need to go crazy counting calories, but I do believe that for the most part, it's simple math: calories in/calories out. Your needs will likely be different than mine, and mine are different sometimes daily, depending on activity level, time of the year, and other circumstances. In general, I aim for 1,600 calories a day, broken down to around 33% each for protein, fat, and carbohydrates (mostly from fiber).

Get yourself an activity tracker (I love my fitbit!) and sign up for one of the many free apps where you can record everything that you eat and drink (MyFitnessPal is the best, in my opinion).

You may be surprised by how much you consume and how little you move. Plus, keeping a food diary is an excellent way to see how foods affect you.

Let's get that out of the way first, so we can move onto the good stuff.

Try to stay away from gluten, even if you don't have celiac disease. Why? There are a few reasons. Today's modern wheat (where most of us get our gluten from- wheat is in so many more products than is obvious) isn't what it was even 50 years ago. It was genetically changed to increase crop yields. William Davis, MD, author of *Wheat Belly*, experimented on himself. He compared his blood sugar after a day of eating ancient wheat (einkorn) bread, and after a day of eating modern wheat bread. Not only did his blood sugar base of 84 mg/dl just about double (167 mg/dl) after eating the modern wheat (compared to the moderate rise to 110 mg/dl with the ancient wheat), he also suffered nausea, fitful sleep, and was unable to think straight for 36 hours.

I myself just returned from a vacation where I fully exercised my 80/20 rule. I may have even flipped it. Gluten was in the beer I drank and in many of my meals. It took five days to recover from a five-day vacation. I was bloated and had a heartburn feeling for days after returning from vacation.

If that's not enough to make you quit the wheat, there's more. It's an appetite stimulant. Much like sugar (more on this later), it makes you want more and more. Much like a drug. Indeed, "exorphins from gluten have the potential to generate euphoria [and] addictive behavior." (*Wheat Belly*) Gluten breaks down in the gut into opioid compounds (gluteomorphins) that trigger the same receptors in the brain as opiate (ie heroin) drugs. (*The Bulletproof Diet*)

Gluten is also inflammatory; an antinutrient. Your body sees it as a toxin. This leads to digestive issues (hello bloat), and an immune response. Your body may begin attacking itself trying to kill the toxic invader. *(The What When Wine Diet)* Inflammation is a risk factor involved in illnesses ranging from colds to cancer, arthritis, heart disease, cognitive decline, and psychiatric and neurological diseases. Guess what? The next two items on my stay-away list, sugar and processed foods, cause the same response.

Sugar. Like wheat, it is everywhere. Like wheat, it is addictive and leads to overconsumption. It's inflammatory, causing hormonal and metabolic dysregulation. And it disrupts gut bacteria balance. (*The Whole 30*) Why is a healthy gut so important? Like Hippocrates said, "All disease begins in the gut." An unhealthy gut can lead to diabetes, obesity, rheumatoid arthritis, autism spectrum disorder, depression, and chronic fatigue syndrome. (www.chriskresser.com) Skip the sugar (and the wheat) and keep the gut healthy!

Sugar and wheat are main components in many processed foods. And you should stay away from them for their double-whammy effect. Processed, pre-packaged foods also tend to contain chemicals and other antinutrients that our bodies don't recognize as food. Generally, their fiber content is low (we love fiber!), and they are flat-out wasted calories. I believe that when people lose weight from low-carb and Paleo diets, it's often because they have eliminated wheat and sugar found in the processed foods that they are now avoiding.

The last things you may want to avoid are corn and soy. They are two other crops that are being messed with, and soy can wreak havoc on some women's hormones. If you aren't soy intolerant, go ahead and eat it. But you can get plant-based proteins elsewhere.

That's what I want you to stay away from. Now the good stuff:

1. Lentils (and other beans, AKA PULSES)

Pulses. I love them so much that I named this plan for them. I started eating lentils and refried beans in earnest after reading *The 4-Hour Body* and *The 20/20 Diet*. Like Cynthia Sass, MPH, RD, states in *Slim Down Now*, "Pulses are the single most underrated superfood."

What's so great about pulses? Where do I even begin? For starters, as a complex carbohydrate, they contain a lot of fiber. Remember, we love fiber! Tanya Zuckerbrot, MS, RD, in *The F-Factor Diet*, found that "women who doubled their fiber intake from 12 to 24 grams per day cut their calorie absorption by 90 calories daily." Fiber acts like a sponge, adding bulk to food, and making you feel fuller longer. Plus, as a soluble fiber, pulses reduce belly fat.

That's just the beginning. They are "protein-dense: [the] single most concentrated source of plant-based protein in the world." (*Bean by Bean a cookbook*, by Crescent Dragonwagon) They contain no cholesterol, and they are low in fat. Not only that, but the polyphenolics in beans aid in assimilating LDL cholesterol and rendering it harmless.

The *Slim Down Now* plan suggests that you eat a pulse serving in at least one meal a day. I agree. The reasons why (listed in *Slim Down Now*):

- boost calories & fat burning
- burn belly fat
- enhance fullness
- support all-day energy
- protect heart
- lower risk for Type 2 diabetes and cancer

- improve overall nutrient intake
- gluten-free
- don't trigger allergies (like soy can)
- affordable and available

I will also add:

- bean crops tend to use less insecticides
- beans are digested slowly, thus stabilizing blood sugar

Similar to the study referenced above, Sass points to a study where women who added five cups of pulses a week lost weight without cutting calories. Whoa.

The 8 Hour Diet (David Zinczenko) has its own list of reasons to eat pulses (beans, peanuts, and other legumes):

- Powers:
  - boost testosterone, build muscle, help burn fat, regulate digestion
- Contain:
  - fiber, protein, iron, folate, MUFA (monounsaturated fatty acids), vitamin E, niacin, magnesium
- Fight:
  - obesity, muscle loss, wrinkles, cardiovascular disease, colon cancer, heart disease, high blood pressure

"Beans, beans, they're good for your heart..." If you're worried about what this song says happens next (gas), up your water intake. And go into it slowly, adding small amounts of pulses (and fiber) every day. Some versions of the song end with "So eat your beans with every meal." If not every meal, every day.

EAT YOUR PULSES!

I like to have lentils or non-fat "refried" beans with my breakfast eggs. Black beans are great thrown into a salad. Kidney beans in chilis. Cannellini beans in a cassoulet. Fava beans in a cold cucumber and tomato salad. Pulses are so versatile! Oh, and how about hummus (chickpea dip)?

Lentils cook up in about 15 minutes. (Lentils also happen to cause less gastrointestinal distress than other legumes.) You can buy any bean canned. Just be sure to rinse them well before eating or cooking with them to reduce the sodium content. I buy my beans dry and cook them in a digital pressure cooker. This saves money and sodium. And cooking in the pressure cooker eliminates overnight soaks. You can have beans ready in a little over an hour.

No excuses. Eat. Your. Pulses.

2. Avocados, olive oil, and other plant fats

These are MUFAs. Monounsaturated Fatty Acids. They are healthy fats found in many plants. Examples of MUFAs are oils, nuts and seeds, avocados, olives, and, wait for it, dark chocolate. I'll concentrate on the oils, avocados, olives and chocolate here since I believe that nuts deserve their own section. One caveat- watch your portions. These are fats, and at 9 calories per gram, the calories pile up quickly.

The *Flat Belly Diet* includes eating a MUFA at every meal as one of their rules. It's a good rule that I use as a guide. Why? Here are a few reasons to add MUFAs to your daily diet:

- they fight belly fat, heart disease, Type 2 diabetes, high blood pressure, and cancer

- they are packed with nutrients and antioxidants

- they fill you up fast, and keep you feeling full longer

For oils, choose olive oil, extra virgin, and (in my opinion) from Italy. This tends to be green in color with a fruity flavor. Drizzle it on salads and vegetables, dip gluten-free bread into it, and cook with it (moderate heat). I use the good stuff raw, and cook with a less expensive brand.

Other oils to consider are sesame oil, avocado oil, walnut, and flaxseed oil. These are best used cold. Grab peanut oil for cooking. Or coconut oil (more on that soon...).

I eat about a half of an avocado a day. Usually ¼ with breakfast, and the other ¼ at lunch in a salad or on a sandwich, or in the afternoon as a snack. And guacamole. I prefer the Haas avocado, but whatever kind you prefer, buy them unripe and when they give to a squeeze, you can cut into them. Tip: store them with the pit (in the refrigerator)- it will keep them from browning.

Oh, and the reason for eating avocados (other than guacamole):

they are a MUFA that is high in cancer-fighting carotenoids.

Olives. They aren't just good for their oil. They are high in Vitamin E, which is an antioxidant that protects cell membranes and reduces inflammation. (Remember- inflammation is bad bad bad).

I love snacking on Spanish olives (the ones stuffed with pimentos), and still will eat black olives off of my finger-tips like I did when I was a kid. Throw them in salads. They also add a unique flavor to stews and sauces. Oh, and tapenade- a condiment mix of olives, oil, and seasonings. Experiment with all of the gorgeous varieties of olives at your supermarket's salad bar, and start incorporating more olives into your life.

Dark chocolate. Do you really need me to tell you the reason why you should eat dark chocolate? I'm going to anyway. Not only is it a MUFA, but it is also a source of resveratrol. (What's so good about resveratrol? Oh, just that it has cancer-fighting properties, is an anti-inflammatory, increases energy levels, and lowers blood sugar.) So yes, I am telling you that dark chocolate is a health food. (Just like wine...)

Keep your portions small. One piece (approximately 45 calories) of dark chocolate, or three cocoa dusted almonds (also about 45 calories), totally satisfies. Or a small handful of dark chocolate chips. Or a gluten-free cookie with dark chocolate chips... Just make sure you are eating dark chocolate with at least 60% cacao.

2.5 Coconut Oil

Coconut oil is a very special plant fat. It is predominantly a saturated fat. Saturated in the form of MCTs (medium chain triglycerides). Most fats are LCTs (long chain triglycerides). What's so great about being an MCT? Some studies have shown that subjects experienced an increase in thermogenesis for a short time after eating MCTs (this does not happen with LCTs). They are absorbed quickly and sent right to the liver, thus being burned as fuel almost entirely. This process may stimulate metabolism. MCTs can boost brain power, assist in fat loss, and make the gut less hospitable to bad bacteria (recall what Hippocrates said about keeping the gut healthy).

I buy coconut oil in bulk. It's my cooking oil of choice for omelets, and any Asian or Hispanic or Indian dish. I use it if I am baking a vegan dessert. I've even begun brushing my teeth with it. (It is an amazing tooth whitener!) And it's the base for my lip balms. (More on that under Smoke & Mirrors.)

Spend the extra and get organic, unrefined coconut oil. By the way, coconut oil is solid at room temperature; if you've never purchased it before, don't look for a clear liquid oil (unless you want the fractionated coconut oil)- it is solid and white.

3. Walnuts, almonds, and other nuts (even peanuts, which are actually a legume)

All of these are MUFAs, like the plant fats above. So they are good for all of the reasons why plant fats are good. They have a few other outstanding properties:

- protein
- fiber
- vitamin E
- magnesium
- muscle builders, craving fighters, and help to reduce wrinkles (!)

I love love love nuts and nut butters, and unless you are allergic to them, I bet you do, too. I buy them in bulk (shelled, unsalted, raw or roasted) and store them in the refrigerator. They are great to snack on (watch serving sizes- they are still a fat and those calories add up), and I love using them (walnuts and almonds in particular) to add crunch to salads where I used to use croutons.

In addition to salads, I use almonds for cooking (with green beans or asparagus), and in baking (almond flour). They, and hazelnuts, also go really well with dark chocolate. And almond butter is terrific. Almonds contain vitamin E and magnesium, and can also help us feel full.

Another nut that is great as a butter is the cashew. I like to think of them as kind of a fancy peanut, and I snack on them like I snack on peanuts. Like peanuts, they work really well in Asian and Indian recipes.

I generally reserve macadamia nuts and pistachios for snacking (especially pistachios as they have the least amount of calories of all nuts), but they both are great with fish and chicken.

Pecans and walnuts may be my favorite nuts. Both are terrific on salads, and both are excellent in baked goods (gluten-free brownies or chocolate chip cookies, anyone?). They go into my oatmeal. I use them in pesto recipes. Walnuts are a particular standout because they are chock full of Omega-3s, a PUFA (polyunsaturated fatty acid). Omega-3s are important for metabolism. In addition, they help with inflammation (there's that word again), mental health, cell growth, and blood clotting. Besides, walnuts are just really yummy.

4. Salsa

I eat salsa everyday. Sometimes at all three meals. It goes with my eggs and avocado at breakfast. I'll have it with a turkey burger at lunch. And it's great on a baked potato. Yes, salsa isn't just for tortilla chips! (Although salsa and chips are a great go-to if you're at a party and the rest of the dips look suspect.)

In general, salsa has about 20 calories per two-tablespoon serving. Good-for-you tomatoes are the base. Flavorful onions, peppers, and herbs and spices are prominent. Salsas come in mild, medium and hot. Some are extra hot. Some have corn. Some have beans. Some have peaches or mangoes. You can make your own, but I haven't been able to perfect mine yet, so I am still purchasing it pre-made. If you do the same, look for ones that are organic, and/or have minimal salt and sugar. Salsas that you find in the refrigerated area (deli usually) of the grocery store are generally better than the ones you find in the Mexican food isle. Mix it up. Try different brands and flavors. And enjoy!

5. Eggs

Even if I didn't raise chickens, I would still eat eggs. They are inexpensive (even if you don't raise chickens), versatile, delicious, and, oh yeah, full of protein. Eggs are good sources of vitamins A, E, and B_{12}. Also iron, zinc, phosphorus, and potassium.

Eggs help you to feel fuller longer, so they are an excellent choice for breakfast. On the days that I do eat breakfast, I am usually eating eggs in the form of an omelet. I serve it with avocado and salsa, and maybe a little cottage cheese and center cut bacon, and any leftover veggies from dinner the night before.

I also like to make a clutch of hardboiled eggs to have on hand for afternoon snacking. One egg with a little salt is super easy and super satisfying, but you can do so much more. Remove the yolk (I give the yolk to my dog) and fill the center with chopped avocado or guacamole, hummus or salsa. Have this with a gluten-free cracker. This should hold you over until dinner.

Don't ignore eggs for dinner. When I have extra eggs, which is usually in the Spring when I have tons of asparagus, I make asparagus fritattas. A slice over salad is a perfect meal, which can be served either hot or cold.

Eggs, "the perfect food."

6. Chicken, fish, and other lean meat

Notice that I said "lean." I try to keep my protein from lean cuts of meat. Do I enjoy Steak Night at the Club? Yes, yes I do. But even then I go for leaner cuts of beef, like a filet mignon or sirloin. Still, these have more than twice as much fat as lean poultry.

Again, notice that I said "lean." Unless it's the white meat from a chicken or turkey, you are getting about the same amount of fat as from a piece of beef. And "the other white meat," pork: same thing. Unless it's the tenderloin, you are getting way too much fat (more than 90 grams of fat in cured pork!).

Yes. You can lose weight eating a high-fat, high-protein, no-carb diet. But tell me how you feel. Personally, if I get too much saturated fat (what is found in animal fats), I feel sluggish and get pains in my upper gut. However, when I am getting protein from lean sources (and my fat from plants), I feel a heck of a lot better.

We eat chicken about twice a week. The various ways to prepare it are endless. We grill it in the summertime, slow-cook it in the wintertime. Stewed, broiled, baked, stir-fried. Almost every cuisine has chicken recipes. And almost every restaurant has chicken entrees.

Once or twice a week I'll have a lean turkey burger for lunch. Usually over a bed of romaine lettuce with a little goat cheese, walnuts, and tomatoes. Yum!

I don't prepare a lot of fish at home, but I encourage you to if you don't mind stinking up your kitchen (my excuse). Fish is what I gravitate towards when I go out to eat, because I know I need more of it. It's good for your heart, and usually has a fraction of the calories of even lean poultry. Grilled is the best way to go (watch sauces). Or, have it my favorite way: sushi and sashimi!

7. Vegetables (leafy and other greens, plus the rest of the rainbow)

"Eat your vegetables!" Eat them at every meal. The reasons to are as varied and wonderful as vegetables themselves:

- neutralize free radicals (those buggers that accelerate the aging process)
- vitamins A, C, K
- folate and beta-carotene
- calcium and magnesium
- fiber to fill you up to keep you regular
- fight cancer, heart disease, stroke, obesity, and osteoporosis

How can you get your vegetables at every meal?

- spinach omelet for breakfast
- asparagus omelet for breakfast
- omelet with peppers for breakfast
- salsa
- salads for lunch or dinner with lots of leafy greens, tomatoes, mushrooms, beans
- bunless turkey burger over a bed of iceberg or romaine lettuce for lunch or dinner
- steamed or grilled asparagus or broccoli with chicken for dinner
- stir-fried veggies with shrimp for dinner

That's just the beginning. Experiment. Try a new vegetable every week. Grow a new vegetable every year if you plant a garden (something we all should be doing, even if it's a small windowbox garden with one tomato plant and basil).

Try to purchase and eat vegetables when they are in season and you can get them locally. If this isn't possible, frozen is your next best choice.

Some of my favorite vegetables (in no particular order) are:

- asparagus
- broccoli
- beets
- kohlrabi
- peppers
- mushrooms
- tomatoes (even though they are technically a fruit)
- spinach
- romaine
- carrots

These just need to be cooked (steamed, grilled, stir-fried) and then topped with a sprinkle of your seasoning of choice, and maybe a little butter.

Most vegetables are super low in calories, so they are almost "free" foods. The complete opposite of empty calories, they are nutrient-rich, giving you a lot (nutritional benefits) for a little (calories). Try to base your meals on vegetables and build upon them; make them the largest portion on your plate.

8. Apples and berries and other fruits (including raisins and prunes)

Like veggies, try to eat fruits and berries when they are in season. Unlike veggies, fruits are not meant for free-for-alls, since they do contain sugar. (We don't like sugar, remember?) But there are still so many reasons to love them, and to eat them every day. Here's why:

- fiber!
- antioxidants and vitamin C
- fight against heart disease, cancer, and obesity
- delicious!

I aim for one or two servings of fruits a day. Any more than that, and it's just way too much sugar. Too much sugar leads to weight gain and a host of other ailments. Have you ever had smoothies for breakfast only to find that you are starving by mid-morning and you're gaining weight? Yep. Sugar.

So how do I get the balance of enough-but-not-too-much?

- If I am not having eggs for breakfast, I'll have oatmeal. I'll add berries or an apple, some walnuts, and then will swirl in some Greek yogurt. A sprinkle of cinnamon and it's a filling and delicious start to my day.
- mango salsa
- cranberry chutney
- grapes in chicken salad
- pork in a cherry sauce
- pineapple chicken
- standing in front of the refrigerator eating a handful of just-

picked blueberries

- Bruce feeding me raspberries from the garden, baby-bird style

I also really like prunes and raisins and other dried fruits. Keep these to a minimum, because the sugar in them is really concentrated. But they go a long way. And they pack a good flavor punch. Raisins with peanut butter on a celery stick, and prunes with peanut butter on a gluten-free cracker are awesome afternoon snacks. I make a few dinners with raisins (they plump up in curries and other stews), and prune rice is so surprisingly delicious!

Plus: <u>WINE!</u>

Ah, the part you were waiting for! (Or did you skip 1-8 and come right here?)

I drink wine every day. I'm no wine snob, but I have also put my box-wine drinking days behind me. Do I drink for the buzz? No. Do I drink for the taste? Yes. And now that I know about all of the health benefits of wine, I drink it for all of those, too.

Plus, wine does not make you gain weight.

Let me say that again: WINE DOES NOT MAKE YOU GAIN WEIGHT.

In fact, it can be part of a weight reduction plan.

Here is where I will say, if you don't already enjoy your red, white, or rose, there's no need to pick up the bottle. (And of course, stay away if you have any addiction issues.)

Oh, and I'm talking moderation here. Don't wake up and start pounding Chianti, and an entire box of chardonnay after work isn't OK, either. Moderation.

When I lost 35 pounds six years ago, it wasn't because I gave up my nightly glass(es) of wine. I didn't cut back, and I didn't go exclusively red or dry white.

This isn't just some fluke, and in this case, I'm not any different from most of you. You, too, likely won't gain weight if you drink wine, and you, too, can lose weight while drinking it.

There are other real health benefits to this alcoholic grape juice. "Studies consistently link moderate alcohol consumption to longevity and healthy biomarkers, even more so than teetotalers!" (*The What When Wine Diet*, by my idol, Melanie Avalon)

What studies, you say? Let me cite a few for you:

Burns J (1), Crozier A, Lean ME. "Alcohol consumption and mortality: is wine different from other alcoholic beverages?" *Nutr Metab Cardiovasc Dis. 2001 Aug; 11(4) : 249-58.*

red wine does indeed offer a greater protection to health than other alcoholic beverages

attributed to grape-derived antioxidant polyphenolic compounds

Ruf JC(1). "Overview of epidemiological studies on wine, health, and mortality." *Drugs Exp Clin Res. 2003;29(5-6):173-9.*

moderate consumption of wine is more beneficial than that of beer or spirits [and] can lower mortality

wine seems to have a beneficial effect on all causes of mortality

in subjects consuming wine in moderation the risk of mortality from all causes is 20-30% lower than in abstainers

Vasanthi HR (1), Parameswari RP, DeLeiris J, Das DK. "Health Benefits of wine and alcohol from neuroprotection to heart health." *Front Biosci (Elite Ed). 2012 Jan 1;4:1505-12.*

daily moderate wine consumption...significant reductions in all-cause and particularly cardiovascular and neurodegenerative mortality when compared with individuals who abstain

López-Vélez M91), Martínez-Martínez F, Del Valle-Ribes C. "The study of phenolic compounds as natural antioxidants in wine." *Crit Rev Food Sci Nutr. 2003;43(3):233-44.*

Plant phenolics present in fruit...particularly rich in red wine...antioxidant activity

protection against cardiovascular diseases and... cancer

four phenolic compounds of red wine: gallic acid, trans-resveratrol, quercetin and rutin

red wine polyphenols are... significant antioxidants

Bertelli AA(1), Das DK. "Grapes, wine, resveratrol, and heart health." *J Cardiovasc Pharmacol. 2009 Dec;54(6):468-76.*

Mild to moderate drinking of wine, particularly red wine, attenuates the cardiovascular, cerebrovascular, and peripheral vascular risk

wine was also found to increase life span by inducing longevity genes

Tresserra-Rimbau A, Medina-Remón A, Lamuela-Raventós RM, Bulló M,
Salas-Salvadó J, Corella D, Fitó M, Gea A, Gómez-Gracia E, Lapetra J, Arós F,
Fiol M, Ros E, Serra-Majem L, Pintó X, Muñoz MA, Estruch R; PREDIMED Study Investigators. "Moderate red wine consumption is associated with a lower prevalence of the metabolic syndrome in the PREDIMED population." *Br J Nutr. 2015 Apr;113 Suppl 2:S121-30.*

Moderate red wine drinkers have a better lipid profile and lower incidence rates of diabetes, hypertension and abdominal obesity

Queipo-Ortuño MI(1), Boto-Ordóñez M, Murri M, Gomez-Zumaquero JM,
Clemente-Postigo M, Estruch R, Cardona Diaz F, Andrés-Lacueva C, Tinahones FJ."Influence of red wine polyphenols and ethanol

on the gut microbiota ecology and biochemical biomarkers." *Am J Clin Nutr. 2012 Jun;95(6):1323-34.*

Red wine consumption can significantly modulate the growth of select gut microbiota in humans, which suggests possible prebiotic benefits associated with the inclusion of red wine polyphenols in the diet

Renaud S(1), de Lorgeril M. "Wine, alcohol, platelets, and the French paradox for coronary heart disease." *Lancet. 1992 Jun 20:339(8808):1523-6.*

France is paradoxical in that there is high intake of saturated fat but low mortality from coronary heart disease (CHD)

high wine consumption... in France... can reduce risk of CHD by at least 40%

Huntly AL(1). "Grape flavonoids and menopausal health." *Menopause Int. 2007 Dec;13(4):165-9.*

Grape flavonoids do benefit the menopausal women

Yang T(1), Li S(2), Zhang X(3), Pang X(4), Lin Q(1), Cao J(1). "resveratrol, sirtuins, and viruses." *Rev Med Virol. 2015 Oct 19.*

diverse biological roles associated with resveratrol, including anti-oxidant, anti-proliferation, anti-inflammation, anti-cancer, anti-fungal, and antiviral activities

Setzer WN(1). "Lignin-derived oak phenolics: a theoretical

examination of additional potential health benefits of red wine." *J Mol Model. 2011 Aug;17(8):1841-5.*

Lingin-derived phenolic compounds can be extracted from oak barrels during the aging of red wine, and... these compounds may contribute to the health benefits of red wine by their antioxidant, radical-scavenging, or chemopreventive activities... and cardioprotective effects of red wine

Letenneur L(1). "Risk of dementia and alcohol and wine consumption: a review of recent results." *Biol Res. 2004;37(2):189-93*

light to moderate alcohol intake might... reduce the risk of dementia and Alzheimer's disease (AD)

regular light to moderate drinking seemed to be associated with a decreased risk for ischaemic stroke

Are those enough scientific studies on the health benefits of wine for you? It's not only what I have experienced. Scientific. Fact.

And articles, too. With grabbing headlines like "Red Wine Burns Fat And Lowers Blood Pressure, Plus 5 Other Health Benefits For Winos" by Samantha Olson on medicaldaily dot com. By the way, she also cites a study from Oregon State's College of Agricultural Studies.

The most recent article hails from the UK, specifically the University of Reading. And, cheers!, it's singing the praises of champagne. The study shows that drinking one to three glasses of the bubbly per week may "counteract the memory loss associated with ageing, and could help delay the onset of degenerative brain disorders, such as dementia." The University previously published a finding that "two glasses of champagne a day may be good for your heart and circulation and could reduce the risks of suffering from cardiovascular disease and stroke."

To sum it up, the health benefits of wine include:
- increased lifespan
- improved insulin sensitivity (discourages insulin resistance)
- protects the heart from cardiovascular disease
- preventative against metabolic syndrome
- may be preventative against rheumatoid arthritis and neurological diseases like Alzheimer's and stroke
- can positively affect stress and depression
- protective against the common cold

(Thank you, Melanie Avalon, again, for this concise list.)

I like that Roger Corder, in *The Red Wine Diet,* writes of wine in the history of health. He points out that Hippocrates, way back in 400 BC, was using wine as an antiseptic, a diuretic, and a sedative. Galen, a Greek physician of the second century AD, was using wine as medicine. And Louis Pasteur, French chemist, said, "Wine is the healthiest and most hygienic of drinks." Yes!

Great, so wine can help you become and stay healthy. It can also help you to become, and to stay, slim. The proof is in the Pinot. And in study after study. Corder cites a French study of male and female subjects who drank up to six glasses of wine a day and who were slimmer than non-drinkers (and heavier drinkers.)

More studies:

Lieber CS(1). "Perspectives: do alcohol calories count?" *Am J Clin Nutr. 1991 Dec;54(6):976-82.*

Chronic consumption of substantial amounts of alcohol is not associated with the expected effect on body weight.

Isocaloric substitution of carbohydrates by ethanol results in weight loss

Wang et al. "Alcohol Consumption, Weight Gain, and Risk of Becoming Overweight in Middle-aged and Older Women." *Archives of Internal Medicine, 2010;170(5):453.*

Normal-weight women who drink a light to moderate amount of alcohol appear to gain less weight and have a lower risk of becoming overweight and obese than nondrinkers

An inverse association between alcohol intake and risk of becoming overweight or obese was noted... with the strongest association found for red wine, and a weak yet significant association for white wine

Women who did not drink alcohol at all gained the most weight, with weight gain decreasing as alcohol intake increased

How can this be? Let me quote *The What When Wine Diet:*

- calories from alcohol do not act like "normal" calories
- hospitalized alcoholics gained NO weight when 1,800 calories in the form of alcohol was added to their standard diet
- substituting 50% of the patients' daily calories with alcohol yielded weight loss
- alcohol's thermogenic effect is around 20%
- alcohol increases metabolism (can raise basal metabolic rate by around 5%)
- alcohol is burned first before other fuel calories
- alcohol does not easily become body fat as no simple or

practical pathway exists for alcohol to fatty acid conversion
- finally, the resveratrol in wine acts like exercise!

And my final word is my before and after where I am drinking wine in both photos.

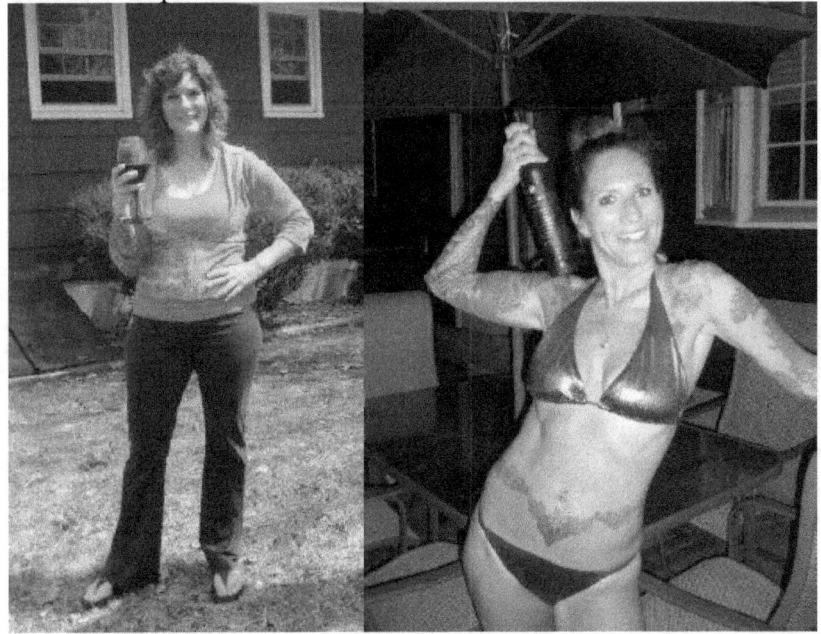

Pulse Fast

You heard it right- the girl who used to scold you for skipping meals (especially breakfast) is now encouraging it. Not every day, unless you are so inclined, but 2-3 days a week. This isn't starvation; it isn't even fasting; this is Intermittent Fasting, a fast (ha) way to lose weight- and more!

There are many different ways to fast intermittently, but the way that I do it is called the Leangains Method, developed by Martin Berkhan. This calls for 14-16 (14 for women, 16 for men) hours of fasting on fasting days. If you sleep for eight of those hours, you are left with a mere 6-8 hours of not eating. For me, this means having a snack and my last glass of wine at 9:00 pm, skipping breakfast, then having lunch at noon. Not bad, right? I have been known to go up to 18 hours, which is fine. After 24-72 hours, you are just plain starving yourself.

What is so magical about this 14-24 hours of fasting? In this time, "the amount of freed-up fatty acids substantially increases" (*What When Wine*) and the body becomes very efficient at cycling fat. The body is now using these freed-up fatty acids as its fuel source, instead of glucose (from food). The body may have run out of glycogen after 8-12 hours, but it hasn't run out of fat...

You only need to fast 2-3 days a week to see the benefits of intermittent fasting. However, with continued intermittent fasting, your body will adapt to using fat more than glycogen. (*Intermittent Fasting*, Valerie Childs)

Both Harvey & Marilyn Diamond (in *Fit For Life)* and David Zinczenko (in *The 8 Hour Diet)* talk about our body's natural hormonal cycle. To simplify:

From noon – 8:00 pm, we are eating and digesting

8:00 pm – 4:00 am, we are absorbing and using what we ate

4:00 am – noon, we are eliminating body waste

This almost perfectly follows my plan of not eating from 9:00 pm until noon the next day. For those of you who are perpetual breakfast skippers, embrace this!

I am not naturally someone who likes to skip breakfast- or any meals. I love to eat, and I love breakfast. You might, too, and you might wonder just how I can not have breakfast and not be starving come lunchtime. Here's how I do it:

- I have coffee, and add collagen peptides to it. The caffeine gets me going, and the small number of calories from the collagen will not break my fast

- I drink spicy lemonade (the Master Cleanse recipe of lemon, maple sugar (or stevia), and cayenne pepper) from coffee until lunchtime

- I keep myself busy

- And, on the days that, for one reason or another I just can't go another moment without food, I eat. And I don't beat myself up over it

Another tip: ease into intermittent fasting. Start with once a week for 12 hours. Then twice a week for 12-14 hours. Work up to three times a week for 14-18 hours. You'll find that it gets easier, and you really won't be hungry.

Another misconception about intermittent fasting is that you will lose muscle. Your body produces amino acids for at least 16 hours after eating a meal with protein. (BCAAs- branched-chain amino acids- are particularly good for muscle repair and glucose metabolism.) Yes, if you starve yourself, you will experience muscle-wasting. Starve. For days and weeks. However, you are not starving yourself. So this is not going to happen.

In fact, "fasted exercise may support muscle growth." (*What When Wine*) I haven't fully embraced working out while fasting yet (I only fast on days when I don't have to teach in the morning), but I do intend to since I have done my own workouts at home on fasting days and didn't come close to keeling over.

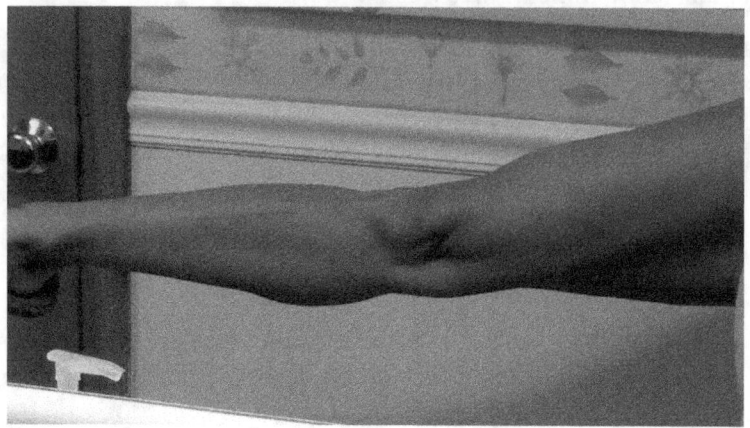

That right there is a 48 year old leg on a body that regularly intermittently fasts. No muscle-wasting there.

So, what are the other benefits of intermittent fasting other than it being an easy way to lose weight quickly?

- metabolic boost
- sharper mental focus
- boosts brain health
- aids in fat loss
- prevents cancer
- builds muscle
- increases resilience
- stress resistance
- prevents chronic disease

- reduces triglycerides
- reduction in blood pressure
- improved insulin responses
- increased lifespan
- immune support/disease resistance
- enhanced exercise
- increased production of Human Growth Hormone (HGH)
- anti-aging at the cellular level

(List compiled from *The What When Wine Diet, The Bulletproof Diet, Intermittent Fasting, and Wheat Belly,* which specifically mentions that eliminating wheat makes intermittent fasting easier.)

Another thing that makes fasting easier? Knowing that you can have a treat meal or day every week. Yup. Continued deprivation doesn't work. I encourage a piece of chocolate and a cookie every day (I'll show you a few of my typical day meal plans later), and I tend to have one meal or one day every week where I go hog-wild and eat whatever I want.

Other experts agree. Dr. Phil, in *The 20/20 Diet,* suggests splurging one or two meals a week. David Zinczenko calls it "cheating" in *The Abs Diet For Women,* and he also encourages doing this one meal a week. Timothy Ferriss takes it a huge step further: he (in *The 4-Hour Body*) insists on one day a week of eating anything and everything that you want. Not only does this keep you on-track the rest of the week, but it also keeps your metabolic rate high.

I also do what Mr. Ferriss does after a treat day: drink something that will encourage gastric emptying (so the crap food is crapped out before it can take hold). Is this scientific? Who knows, but I know that I don't feel as disgusting in the morning if I have a cup of weak senna tea before bed after chowing down on pizza and beer... (Do not do this more than once a week.)

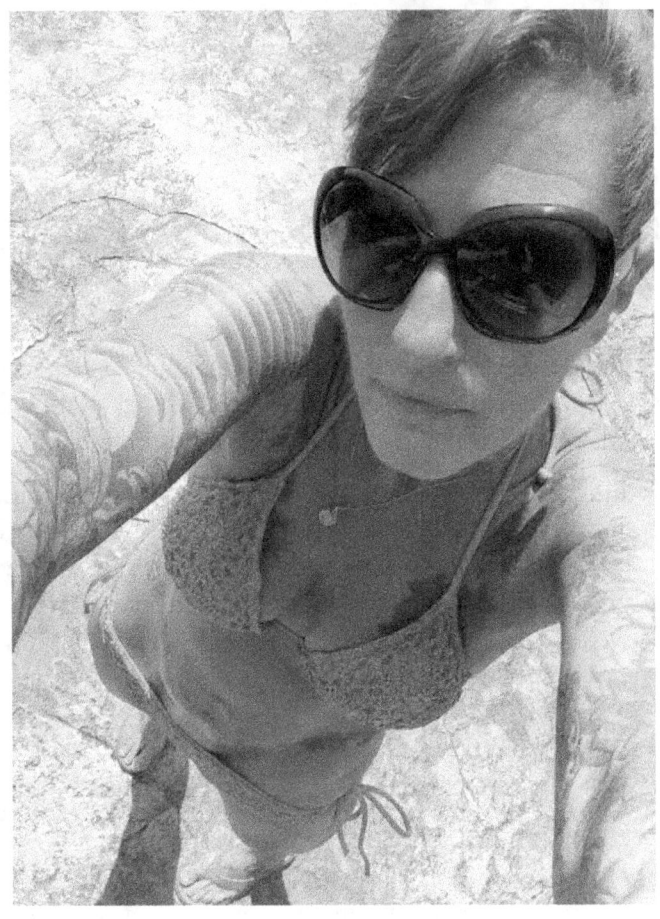

Pulse Supplements

I used to have a cabinet full of vitamins and other supplements. A multi-vitamin, Vitamin C, other herb and mineral blends purported to help me lose weight, feel more energetic, not get sick... I now know that most of these pills were only working on making my wallet lighter. The bioavailability of most supplements is minimal, and that's when you are getting what is actually on the label.

Ideally we wouldn't need to supplement our diets, but, as mentioned earlier, today's food just isn't what it was before. Our soil just doesn't have the minerals in it that it used to. And so, from the ground up, literally, we aren't getting what we used to from our food.

There are a few ways that I have decided to supplement my mostly healthy diet.

First, I drink either Maximum Vibrance or Green Vibrance (both from Vibrant Health) every day. Vibrant Health is a Connecticut-based company (like our produce, why shouldn't our supplements also be local- at least for me?), and I like how their products are gluten-free, vegan, with no proprietary blends.

Green Vibrance is the most award winning nutritional supplement. It contains plant based micro-nutrition, antioxidant life preservers, immune support, adaptogens, skeletal support, fiber, liver support, enzymes and tonics, and probiotics. (Find all ingredients at www.vibranthealth.com) So what are the benefits? Support for digestion and gastrointestinal function, healthy circulation, clearance of waste products of metabolism, detoxification, neurological health, cardiovascular function, normal blood sugar and cholesterol, immunity, healthy bones, plus more energy and resistance to oxidative changes associated with aging. I drink Green Vibrance on days that I am not fasting.

Maximum Vibrance has all of the above, plus it is a multivitamin and protein powder- a true meal replacement. In fact, it is often how I break my fast on days that I am intermittent fasting, since its protein is plant-based BCAAs. It's also what I take on vacation with me. (Again, ingredients can be found on the Vibrant Health website. Again, full disclosure.) Maximum Vibrance isn't just a superfood- it's "The World's 1st Futurefood™." Feel free to drink it every day!

The second supplement that I take daily are Collagen Peptides from Vital Proteins. Peptides are short chain amino acids derived from collagen protein. Why take them? They:

- promote youthful skin, healthier hair, and stronger nails

- help keep bones healthy and strong

- support joint health

- contribute to a balanced diet and help maintain weight

- support healthy inflammation response due to overexercise

- natural glycine improves sleep quality

I stir this "100% Natural Anti-Aging Dietary Supplement" into my coffee every morning. You can also mix it with cold drinks, or even into recipes. (More ideas, plus supplement facts on the Vital Proteins website: www.vitalproteins.com)

(By the way, I am an affiliate for both of these companies, but that isn't why I promote them. I just love them and how I look and feel taking them. You can purchase them at some health food stores, online on their websites, or through my website, www.yolarates.com/Shop.html, where you can get a discount.)

In addition to my "green drinks" and collagen, I take krill oil and turmeric for my old dancer's joints, and zinc, selenium, chromium, and gigartina for my fibromyalgia and hypothyroidism (as needed when my body is under stress). You may need to occasionally supplement your supplements differently.

Pulse Exercise

Exercise may only be 20% of the equation, but that's still twenty percent. You need to move your body to lose weight, maintain a healthy weight, and to stay youthful and healthy. However, you do not need to workout like a maniac to reap these benefits. In fact, for many of us, less is more.

A few years ago, before I understood this, I was frustrated because I was teaching a dozen fitness classes a week, plus hitting the treadmill almost daily, and doing exercise DVDs on days that I didn't teach. And yet, not only was I not losing weight, but I was gaining it. I was by no means overweight, but I wasn't comfortable in my own skin, and frankly, not being in good shape is bad for business.

And then I read something in *The Thyroid Diet Revolution* (Mary J. Shomon); "Don't exercise too much!" She explains that we do need moderate activity, but that excessive exercise can create stress and adrenal fatigue. Ah, that explained it.

Dave Asprey (in *The Bulletproof Diet*) goes further to say, "Your body responds to rigorous exercise as it does to any other stressor: by increasing cortisol levels in your body."

Just what is cortisol, and why is too much of it so bad? Cortisol is a hormone that can increase blood sugar, suppress the immune system, and decrease bone formation. If it is elevated for an extended amount of time, it can lead to weight gain and muscle loss. Ack.

So, too much exercise can be stressful, but I do recommend staying active and participating in organized exercise. Moderate exercise has been shown to improve bone density and mood, increase insulin sensitivity and lean muscle, decrease inflammation, and lead to a better night's sleep.

Everyone is different, and I tell clients that they need to find what kind of exercise they and their bodies like. Often this means looking back at sports you played as a kid, or dance classes you took after school. If it doesn't feel like exercise- a chore- you will be much more apt to stick with the program. (Just don't go overboard! And don't think that just because you've worked out in the morning that you can sit on the couch all afternoon and stuff your face all night.)

For me, it's been dance. My parents started me in ballet classes before my fourth birthday, and I fell in love. Don't ask me to run a marathon (although I did finish a 5K two years ago), and don't ask me to go to Cross Fit with you. My body just isn't into these activities.

And remind me to say "No" to teaching too many high-intensity classes a week. This just recently happened to me- I took on more than my body likes, and took out what it loves. After a summer of teaching my YoLarates™ barre class three times a week at night, the Fall class session started and I was only teaching it once a week, but was teaching a circuit-training class and a Zumba® Fitness class instead. In the summer, I was burning less calories and taking less steps (besides the kind of exercise I was doing, I also spend countless hours sitting poolside in the summer), and yet with the added activity, I added five pounds to my frame. My body was under stress...

On the flip side, I was one of the few people who lost weight over Thanksgiving. Why? Because I gave my body a break. No classes. No intense exercise. Less is more for me.

What works for me, and what might work for you, is a blend of low-impact/low-intensity cardio (in the form of Zumba®Gold) and bodyweight training (in the form of my YoLarates™ barre class). If you don't have access to classes locally, you can look for workouts on YouTube, see what you like, and then purchase the DVDs. Exercise is highly individual. And you need to do it; just not too much!

Pulse Smoke and Mirrors

I honestly want to focus on how I (and my clients) feel. For me, it really is about being as healthy as I can as I get older. But I ain't gonna lie- I wanna look good, too. I'm willing to bet that you are, too.

Eating right and exercising properly generally will make you look good, in addition to getting you healthy. But there's nothing wrong with helping things along.

I'm not encouraging plastic surgery. If you want to embrace Botox and silicone, I won't judge. But that's not for me. I'm trying to put up a graceful fight.

Botox = Bangs (to cover forehead lines)

Breast enhancements = Victoria's Secret Miracle Bra

Lip injections = Lara's Luscious Lip Balm Cinnamon

Liposuction = YoLarates™

I call this "smoke and mirrors."

The first step is taking care of your skin. I do this from the inside by taking collagen, but also topically. Our skin is our largest organ, so it makes sense to take care of it, and to be heedful of what we put on it.

In the (not so distant) past, I would try any and all forms of anti-aging potions, no matter what the ingredients were. Similar to my experience with "nutritional" supplements, in most cases, I was merely cleaning out my cash cache. More times than not, whatever it was that I was using, didn't live up to its claims to banish wrinkles, promote soft and smooth skin, or to reduce cellulite.

Plus, almost all contained toxic ingredients that weren't only wreaking havoc on my skin, but also on my hormones and other body systems.

How's that? As mentioned, our skin is our largest organ. Anything we put on it is absorbed in 20 seconds. Which means, even if it's just a facial cleanser, it's going inside.

Take a moment here: go read the ingredients on your facial cleanser.

Scary, huh?

Scarier still is if you start reading the ingredients of your make-up. Something that sits on (IN) your skin all day.

Your body lotions.

Sunscreens.

And the scariest for me yet: lipstick. Not only is this on the sensitive skin of your lips, but it's right there, at your mouth. For you to eat.

When I starting thinking about this, I freaked out a little. My facial cleanser now is coconut oil. That's it. I smear my face with a healthy tablespoon of it, massage it in, then wipe it off with a hot, wet washcloth.

And, I started making my own lip balm. And, because I like pretty as well as functional, I added shimmer to it. Glittery mica (a mineral) is how I safely do this. For mild plumping and a sweet smell, I use peppermint or cinnamon essential oils. These are on a nourishing and natural base of coconut oil, shea butter, beeswax and vitamin E.

I think this lip balm is so fabulous that I have started selling it at Annalisa Studio and through my website, www.larafoldvari.com

I didn't stop with lip balm, and you shouldn't either. My deodorant is all-natural (Lavanila). And my cellulite-fighting oil. So is my shampoo and conditioner. Eye cream and facial lotion. Body lotion, too. (I make all of these myself.)

Body lotion that I have made bronzed and glittery (with mica).

Bronzed and glittery. AKA smoke and mirrors.

First the bronze. Or the tan. I'm a sun-worshipper. Not only because it's relaxing. Or for the Vitamin D (go outside and grab 15 minutes of sunshine a day to get your dose- even if it means just driving to work without your sunglasses on). It's for the tan. I look so much better when I am bronzed. I look healthier. I look more toned. And I look younger.

If you aren't into subjecting yourself to skin cancer (do still try to get your 15-minutes of unprotected sunshine in daily- even if it's just enjoying some quality time with your fur-friend in a sunny window), there are excellent self-tanners on the market that will give you a faux glow. Look for more natural brands, such as bareMinerals and Vita Liberata.

bareMinerals also makes an excellent mineral foundation. It almost makes your skin look flawless- and it's good for it!

Don't stop with your skin. Thin, frizzy hair can show your age and health status, too. Keep it clean. Keep it conditioned. And don't be afraid to add glitter. (Yup. I add a pinch of mica to my hair gel.)

Graying hair is another matter. I've been blessed since I just have a few annoying silver streaks. Once I'm more than 25% gray, I will become a bottle brunette. And you can bet that I will be finding the most natural way to do this.

A huge way to add or subtract years is with your mouth. Not just your lips, but your teeth. Taking care of your teeth is something that you should've been doing since you were able to stand on your own, but, if you haven't, then start now.

Floss. At least once a day. And brush. At least once a day. Toothpaste is another one of those nasties that is full of chemicals that we don't need. Try to find a natural one.

Or, make your own. I now brush with a crazy mix of coconut oil and activated charcoal. It looks horrifying while I am brushing, but the result is that my teeth are cleaner and whiter than they've ever been- chemical-free.

I'm also skipping nail polish now. My nails are healthy because of my diet and the collagen, so all they need is to be kept clean and buffed.

Finally, dress and accessorize to accentuate or hide. Even though I am almost 50 years old, I have no shame in wearing fashionably torn jeans, graphic tees, and high-heels. No matter your age, there is no reason to dress like a frump. You don't have to spend a million dollars, and you don't have to look like you just stepped off a runway, but do take care of what you cover your healthy body with.

This also means to wear clothes that fit. Jeans that are bagging off of you are just as bad as crop-tops on big bellies. Check your mirror before you leave the house. Please.

And don't forget the glitter!

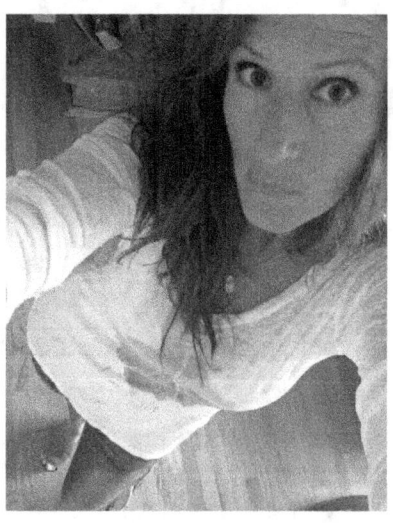

Pulse Lists

At the grocery store:

Fruits
Avocados
Apples
Bananas
Berries (blueberries, raspberries, strawberries, blackberries)
Grapefruit
Lemons
Limes
Oranges
Pears
Tomatoes
Frozen fruits and vegetable mixes

Veggies

Garlic
Cucumber
Onions
Lettuce (Romaine, Boston, Iceberg)
Spinach
Kale
Asparagus
Broccoli
Celery
Potatoes
Sweet Potatoes
Squash (Summer, Zucchini, Spaghetti, Acorn)
Mushrooms

Pulse

Green Beans
Beets
Bell peppers (red, green, yellow, orange)
Herbs (basil, cilantro, parsley, mint, chives, rosemary)

Meats

Boneless, skinless chicken breasts
Pork chops
Steaks (Porterhouse, sirloin, tenderloin, flank)
Lean ground beef (at least 90% lean)
Lean ground turkey meat (99% lean)
Turkey or chicken kielbasa (no nitrates, please)
Other turkey or chicken sausages
White fish (halibut, cod, red snapper)
Tuna- sushi grade steaks
Bacon, center cut

"Dairy"

Almond milk
Coconut milk
Eggs
Fat-free Greek yogurt (Fage brand)
Low-fat sour cream (Daisy brand)
Low-fat cottage cheese (Friendship brand)
Farmer's cheese
Butter, from grass-fed cows
Goat or sheep milk cheese

Grains

Gluten-free flour (Bob's Red Mill 1-to-1 baking flour)

Pulse

Brown rice (short, long, Basmati, Jasmine)
Quinoa
Millet
Amaranth
Buckwheat
Gluten-free pasta
Gluten-free bread (Udi and Schar)
Gluten-free tortilla wraps
Rolled oats
Cream of Rice

Herbs & Spices

Hungarian sweet paprika
Cumin
Madras curry powder
Crushed red pepper
Spike seasoning
Fines Herbes
Herbs de Provence
Nutmeg
Cinnamon
Vanilla extract

Fats (oils & nuts)

Almonds, walnuts, pecans, cashews, peanuts
All-natural nut butters
Powdered peanut butter
Extra virgin olive oil
Coconut oil
Shredded coconut

Canned goods

Stock & broth- low-sodium and gluten-free
Beans! (black, pinto, cannellini, chick peas, lentils, kidney)
Crushed or chopped tomatoes
Tomato paste
Olives
White tuna in water
Artichoke hearts
Low-sodium soups

Miscellaneous

Mustards
Salsa
Honey
Maple syrup
Stevia
Vinegar (apple, wine, rice, balsamic)
Coconut Aminos
Coconut water
Dark chocolate
Wine

Meal Plan- what Lara typically eats on any given day

Breakfast:

One egg
One egg white only
Canadian bacon or lowfat cottage cheese
lentils or black beans or refried beans
salsa
guacamole or avocado slices
gluten-free toast or gluten-free crackers
coffee with stevia, collagen peptides, and coconut milk beverage

OR

Oatmeal with chia seeds, hemp and flax seeds
walnuts
mixed berries, and apple, or raisins or prunes
Greek yogurt
coffee with stevia, collagen peptides, and coconut milk beverage

Lunch:

lettuce, no salad dressing or one tablespoon oil and vinegar
dressing or salt and pepper and herbs of choice
add grilled chicken or a can of tuna, and chickpeas or cannellini
beans
walnuts, salsa, and avocado
cottage cheese or goat or sheep cheese and olives optional
One piece of dark chocolate

OR

Leftovers

Dinner:

chicken breast or thigh, grilled or fish
lentils or black beans or cannellini beans
vegetable of choice (spinach, broccoli, asparagus, squash)

Snacks:

Quest bar (I like to have half and save the other half for another day)
Gluten-free crackers (Crunchmaster are my favorites) or tortilla chips with cottage cheese or guacamole or egg whites or hummus
nuts and fruit
Greek yogurt (Fage non-fat, plain) with gluten-free granola (I like Kind)
veggies (carrots, celery) dipped in light Ranch dressing
Gluten-free chocolate chip cookie (recipe forthcoming)

Drinks:

water
tea
Wine!

On fasting days, skip breakfast and any morning snack and have instead:

coffee with stevia, collagen peptides, and coconut milk beverage
Master Cleanse (lemon, cayenne pepper, maple sugar or stevia)

Pulse

Favorite recipes

There are a few things that I eat all the time that I had to create recipes for because the ones I had found were full of things that I didn't want to load into my body. I'd like to share these with you.

For most recipes, I suggest searching the internet or grabbing a cookbook (I list my favorites in the Bibliography/Suggested Reading section).

I recommend it in my book, _Just a Good Cook..._ and I'll say it again: experiment. Take recipes and tweak them.

I don't much count calories, and unless I am baking, I don't much measure ingredients.
I also won't give you number of servings/recipe; if you want to eat all the guacamole, I won't be the one to stop you.

Pulse

"Refried" Beans

You can get the stuff in the can, but why should you when this is almost as easy, costs a fraction of the canned stuff, and you know what's in it?

One can (rinsed) pinto beans
 or
One cup dry pinto beans, cooked

To taste:

onion and garlic powder
cumin and cayenne pepper
salt and pepper

Add the seasonings and mash into the beans

Pulse

Guacamole

Everyone has their own favorite recipe for guacamole. Here's mine.

One ripe avocado

salt and pepper
garlic powder
cumin
lime juice
hot sauce
fresh cilantro

Add the lime juice, hot sauce and seasonings and mash into the avocado

Pulse

<u>Picadillo</u>

I like to pretend that I'm Cuban. Here's my nod to my non-heritage.

Approximately ½ pound each lean ground turkey and beef
One small onion
Sofrito sauce (made by Goya)
garlic powder
salt and pepper
garlic powder
oregano (dried)
cumin
One can diced tomatoes
One (very) large splash sherry
¼ cup (golden) raisins
¼ cup Spanish olives
One Tablespoon capers
Fresh parsley

Brown the meat, then add the onion and sofrito. Once the onion is soft, add the rest of the ingredients, except for the parsley. Cover and simmer for 15-30 minutes, then garnish with parsley.

Gluten-free Vegan Chocolate Chip Cookies

These aren't low-cal, but they are delicious and very satisfying. And gluten-free. And vegan. And relatively low-sugar. I make a batch, freeze them, and eat one every night. Every. Night.

2 Tablespoons chia seeds, soaked in 6 Tablespoons water
1 cup Bob's Red Mill 1-to-1 baking flour
1 cup gluten-free oats
¼ cup King Arthur Flour gluten-free whole grain flour (or Ancient Grains flour)
½ teaspoon cinnamon
1 teaspoon baking soda
1 teaspoon salt
1 teaspoon vanilla extract
½ cup coconut oil
½ cup apple sauce (unsweetened)
¼ cup Truvia baking sugar
¼ cup Truvia baking brown sugar
1 ½ cups dark chocolate chips (dairy & soy free)
1 cup chopped walnuts

Preheat the oven to 375°

Soak the chia seeds in the water in a small bowl.

Mix the flours, oats, cinnamon, baking soda, and salt in a large bowl.

Add the coconut oil, apple sauce, sugars and the chia seed/water mixture (which should be like a gel by now) to the flour mixture. Mix well, then add the chocolate chips and walnuts.

Use parchment paper or a silicone baking sheet on a cookie sheet.

Pulse

Drop by rounded Tablespoons and bake for about 12 minutes at 375°.

Makes just under 50 cookies.

Let them cool, then store them in the freezer. Eat one every day.

Final Thoughts

There you have it. What I am currently doing to "keep the beat of youth." But it's not just what I am doing. My clients are also doing it and seeing results. Because it's backed by science. I gave you a list of studies in the wine section, but I have a list of books that I also referenced. (They, and other suggested books, are in Appendix I.) Since wine-as-health-food and intermittent fasting are controversial ideas, I felt that I had to give sources and not just my experience with them.

How I take care of myself, and how I coach clients and students, is constantly evolving. Keep current with me on social media at www.facebook.com/larafoldvari, www.facebook.com/yolarates, and on Instagram as larafold. I post a lot of my meals, fitness and nutrition tips, and a weekly Fit Friday video.

And by all means, let me know how YOU do with the *Pulse*!

Cheers!

Appendix I

Bibliography

Asprey, D. (n.d.). *The bulletproof diet: Lose up to a pound a day, reclaim energy and focus, and upgrade your life.* New York: Rodale

Avalon, M. (2015). *The what when wine diet, Paleo and intermittent fasting for health and weight loss.* Los Angeles, CA: Incandescent Expressions

Burroughs, S. (2012). *The master cleanser.* Snowball Publishing

Childs, V. (n.d.). *Intermittent fasting: Simple guide to weight loss, fat loss and improved health : The fat loss and anti aging diet.*

Corder, R. (2007). *The red wine diet.* New York: Avery Pub Group.

Davis, W. (2011). *Wheat belly: Lose the wheat, lose the weight, and find your path back to health.* Emmaus, Penn.: Rodale.

Diamond, H., & Diamond, M. (1985). *Fit for life.* New York, NY: Warner Books.

Dragonwagon, C. (2011). *Bean by bean.* New York: Workman Pub.

Ferriss, T. (2010). *The 4-hour body: An uncommon guide to rapid fat-loss, incredible sex, and becoming superhuman.* New York: Crown Archetype.

Fletcher, A. (2003). *Thin for life.* New York: Houghton Mifflin

Pulse

Company

Hartwig, D. (2015). *Whole 30, The: The Official 30-Day Guide to Total Health and Food Freedom.* London: Hodder & Stoughton General Division.

McGraw, P. (n.d.). *The 20/20 diet: Turn your weight loss vision into reality : 20 key foods to help you succeed where other diets fail.* Los Angeles, CA: Bird Street Books, Inc.

Sass, C. (n.d.). *Slim down now: Shed pounds and inches with real food, real fast.* New York: HarperCollins

Shomon, M., & Shomon, M. (2012). *The thyroid diet revolution: Manage your master gland of metabolism for lasting weight loss.* New York: HarperCollins.

Vaccariello, L. (2009). *Flat belly diet! pocket guide: Introducing the easiest, budget-maximizing eating plan yet!* New York: Rodale.

Zinczenko, D., & Spiker, T. (2007). *The abs diet for women: The six-week plan to flatten your belly and firm up your body for life.* Emmaus, Pa.: Rodale.

Zuckerbrot, T. (2006). *The F-factor diet: Discover the secret to permanent weight loss.* New York: G.P. Putnam's Sons.

Suggested Reading

Acquista, A., & Vandermolen, L. A. (2006). *The Mediterranean prescription: Meal plans and recipes to help you stay slim and healthy for the rest of your life*. New York: Ballantine Books.

Blatner, D. J. (2009). *The flexitarian diet: The mostly vegetarian way to lose weight, be healthier, prevent disease and add years to your life*. New York: McGraw-Hill.

Frankel, B., & Adamson, E. (2010). *The skinnygirl dish: Easy recipes for your naturally thin life*. New York: Simon & Schuster.

Grandhi, B. (2009). *Spice up your life*. Springville, UT: CFI.

Hunn, N. (2011). *Gluten-free on a shoestring: 125 easy recipes for eating well on the cheap*. New York: Da Capo Lifelong.

Maffucci, A. (2015). *Inspiralized: Turn vegetables into healthy, creative, satisfying meals*.

Michaels, J. (2013). *Slim for life: My insider secrets to simple, fast, and lasting weight loss*.

Peláez, A. S. (2014). *The Cuban table: A celebration of food, flavors, and history*.

Reno, T. (2007). *The eat-clean diet cookbook: Great-tasting recipes that keep you lean!* Mississauga, ON: R. Kennedy Pub.

Vaccariello, L., & Sass, C. (2008). *Flat belly diet! cookbook*. Emmaus, PA: Rodale.

William, A. (2015). *Medical medium: Secrets behind chronic and mystery illness and how to finally heal*.

Appendix II

Stuff I love

I have a ton of gadgets that I love. Most can be found on amazon.com. Here's the short list:

1. my spiralizer
2. my digital pressure cooker
3. my NuWave oven
4. my fitbit
5. my iPhone

Beauty Products I love

This list is evolving, but right now, these are some of the products that you can find in my bathroom:

1. bareMinerals Mineral Veil powder
2. itCosmetics eyeliner
3. Vita Liberata self-tanners
4. bareMinerals glimmer eyeshadows (Bare Skin!)
5. Lavanila deodorant
6. Mally eye shadow sticks (Dusk!)

Favorite Apps for my iPhone

Another evolving list:

1. MyFitnessPal
2. fitbit
3. Think Dirty (mind out of gutter: it's for finding toxic beauty products)
4. SparkRecipes
5. Inspiralized
6. Wellness Mama
7. amazon.com

Websites to check out

Yup. Also evolving:

1. **www.sophieuliano.com**
2. **www.vibranthealth.com**
3. **www.vitalproteins.com**
4. **www.yolarates.com**
5. **www.penzeys.com**
6. **www.amazon.com**
7. **www.wellnessmama.com**
8. **www.jenniraincloud.com**

Appendix III

The 3-4-7 Cleansing Detox Jumpstart

Sometimes, especially at the beginning of the year, or before a big event, you need a little extra oomph to flatten your belly, get rid of toxins and other garbage that may be slowing you down and making you feel, and maybe look, like crud. Usually I am an advocate of a slow-and-steady, moderate approach to weight loss, but I'm also not immune to over-indulging and wanting to reverse the effects ASAP. And so, my 3-4-7 Cleansing Detox Jumpstart.

3-day Cleanse

It starts with a 3-day cleanse. Specifically, the Master Cleanse. Naturopath Stanley Burroughs created this lemonade diet in the 1940s to cleanse the system. Every morning starts with drinking salt water (up to one quart of water with two teaspoons of non-iodized sea salt). I have skipped this step, but if you really want to clean yourself out, go for it. Just make sure you don't have any plans that take you far from a toilet...

The lemonade is a much more enjoyable part of the diet. It consists of drinking 5-12 glasses of the lemonade a day. Each glass of the lemonade is made of:

> 2 Tablespoons lemon juice
>
> 2 Tablespoons maple syrup
>
> 1/10 teaspoon cayenne pepper
>
> 10 ounces filtered water

At night, enjoy a glass of laxative tea made from senna.

Burroughs suggested staying on this diet for 10-40 days, and I do know people who have done so successfully, but I believe that we only need three days, and that anything more than that can be dangerous.

If you are lazy, or don't have time, or just don't feel like messing around with making lemonade all day long for three days, you can order Master Cleanse kits. I get mine from Vibrant Health (called Vibrant Cleanse). It includes enough packets to make five glasses of lemonade for three days, plus Himalayan salt and laxative tea. Basically, everything you need for the 3-day cleanse. How easy is that? If you order through my website, www.yolarates.com, you can find a link to Vibrant Health and a code to get 20% off.

4-day Detox

The Cleanse can be followed by a Detox that includes solid food. You won't be totally cleansing like you were on the Cleanse, but you will be continuing to detox. This is four days of consuming the same breakfasts, lunches, and dinners, every day.

Breakfast:

> Don't. Don't break your fast quite yet. You can have a cup of green tea, and if you purchased the Vibrant Cleanse from Vibrant Health, you can also have the packet of Field of Greens that came with the kit. Keep drinking water throughout the morning. (If you have leftover Cleanse ingredients and are hungry, or just can't get down plain water, feel free to make lemonade.)

Lunch:

> Make a protein meal replacement shake from your favorite brand. I use Maximum Vibrance (from Vibrant Health, of course) because it has BCAAs and superfoods, but if you have one that you are in love with, use that. Make sure that it has around 20 grams of protein.

Keep drinking water or lemonade or green tea in the afternoon. If you get hungry (which you may not, after three days of cleansing), have a small piece of fruit (an apple, or a tangerine are my two favorites) or some veggies (I like the crunch from carrots or celery).

Dinner:

> Make a huge salad. Start with romaine and spinach and go from there. Sprinkle with a salt-free seasoning. Add tomatoes and bell peppers. Broccoli and cauliflower. And four ounces of lean protein, like chicken, turkey, or fish. (Vegetarians can have a hardboiled egg; vegans can have tofu.)

Pulse

Keep drinking water or lemonade or green tea until bedtime.

Wake up and repeat for the next three days (for a total of four days).

7-day Jumpstart

You get to eat even more food during the Jumpstart, and, if your system feels OK with it, you can add your pulses and wine now. (Yes!)

Breakfast:

You can continue to hold off on breaking your fast (extending intermittent fasting), or you can have of my two favorite breakfasts.

1. Eggs

   1 large egg and one egg white

   avocado or guacamole

   salsa

   pulse of choice

2. Oatmeal

   ½ cup old fashioned oats

   1 Tablespoon chopped walnuts

   1 Tablespoon plant protein powder, vanilla flavor

   ½ cup berries

Oh, and go ahead and have your coffee with a splash of non-dairy milk, stevia, and collagen peptides. (Or black.)

Keep drinking water, lemonade, or green tea.

Lunch:

Have a big salad. Start with romaine and spinach, add more veggies, and sprinkle with a salt-free seasoning. Top with your lean protein, then throw in a few walnuts or ¼ of an avocado, and your pulse of choice.

Afternoon snack:

> Your favorite protein meal replacement shake, halved. If you get hungry, have a small piece of fruit or veggies.

Keep drinking water, lemonade, or green tea.

Dinner:

> Repeat lunch. Or, have a 4-ounce portion of lean protein with a cup of steamed veggies, sprinkled with salt-free seasoning. Serve with ½ cup brown rice, or quinoa, or lentils.

Enjoy a glass of wine!

Repeat for the next six days. Try to get into the habit of eating the same thing most days. Studies have shown that eating the same foods daily helps in keeping weight off. This is a good habit to get into.

About the Author

Lara Foldvari is 48 years old and counting. She is certified by AFAA and ACE as a Group Fitness Instructor and Personal Trainer, and she is a NASM certified Fitness Nutrition Specialist, as well as a NESTA certified Lifestyle & Weight Management Specialist.

Lara teaches YoLarates™ and Zumba® classes in the Cheshire, CT area. She also trains and coaches clients in fitness and nutrition.

When she isn't teaching, training, or coaching, you can find her floating around her pool (weather permitting), sitting with her chickens (also weather permitting), cooking, creating natural beauty products, reading, or traveling. And always, with a glass of wine in hand.

www.larafoldvari.com

www.yolarates.com

lara@yolarates.com

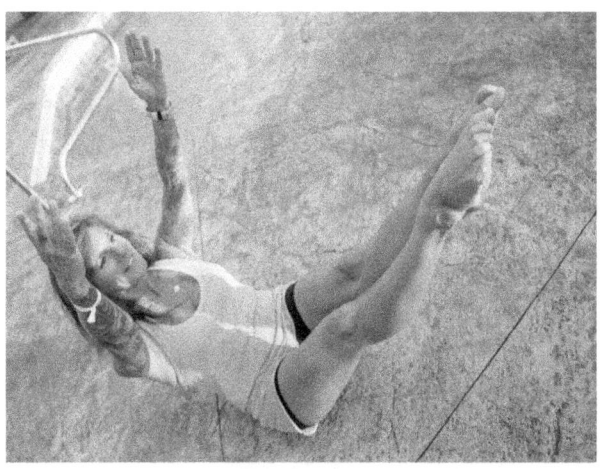